DIABETES TREATMENT:

The Healthiest Way to Enjoy Your Favorite Meals

Copyright ©2023 by **Lori J. Altman**

INTRODUCTION

A chronic health condition called diabetes affects millions of people worldwide. It is a metabolic condition where the body struggles to control blood glucose levels, resulting in elevated glucose levels in the blood (hyperglycemia). A person's general health and life satisfaction may be significantly impacted by the complex condition of diabetes. Many consequences, including as harm to the kidneys, eyes, nerves, and blood vessels, might result from it.

Type 1 and type 2 diabetes are the two most prevalent types of the disease, while there are other varieties as well. When the body's immune system attacks and destroys the insulin-producing cells, type 1 diabetes, an autoimmune illness that commonly manifests in childhood or adolescence, results the pancreas' cells. Contrarily, type 2 diabetes is a metabolic illness that typically manifests in maturity and is brought on when the body develops an insulin resistance or a deficiency.

Diabetes must be managed and monitored carefully throughout one's lifetime. Medication, dietary modifications, and routine blood sugar testing are frequently used as treatments. People with diabetes can live healthy, active lives and lower their risk of complications with adequate management. To better understand and manage this complex disease, however, more research and education are required.

Diabetes continues to be a major public health concern.

CHAPTER ONE

DEFINITION OF DIABETES

Diabetes is a long-term metabolic condition that develops when the body struggles to control blood glucose levels. When the body either produces insufficient insulin or uses it inefficiently, this occurs. The pancreas secretes insulin, a hormone that facilitates glucose uptake into cells for use as fuel. Without adequate insulin, glucose builds up in the blood, resulting in elevated blood sugar levels, which over time may result in a number of health issues. There are two primary varieties of diabetes: Type 1, which is brought on by the immune system of the body attacking and destroying pancreatic insulin-producing cells, and Type 2, which is brought on by a confluence of insulin resistance and decreased insulin production. When your blood glucose, commonly known as blood sugar, is too high, you develop diabetes. Your primary energy source is blood glucose, which is obtained from the food you eat. The pancreas produces the hormone insulin, which facilitates the entry of food-derived glucose into your cells for energy production. Your body occasionally produces insufficient insulin, none at all, or uses it improperly. After that, glucose remains in your circulation and does not enter your cells.

BLOOD TYPES AND DIABETES

Although the connection between blood types and diabetes is not entirely known, various studies have been done to look into the possibility. Key conclusions are as follows:

1. **Type 2 diabetes and blood type A:** According to some research, people with blood type A may be more prone to the disease than people with other blood types. For instance, a study that appeared in the Journal of Clinical Endocrinology and Metabolism indicated that persons with blood type A were more likely than people with blood type O to experience insulin resistance, which is a precursor to type 2 diabetes.

2. **Type 2 diabetes and blood type A:** According to some research, people with blood type A may be more prone to the disease than people with other blood types. For instance, a study that appeared in the Journal of Clinical Endocrinology and Metabolism indicated that persons with blood type A were more likely than people with blood type O to experience insulin resistance, which is a precursor to type 2 diabetes.

3. **Blood type AB and gestational diabetes:** According to some study, women with blood type AB may have a higher risk of developing gestational diabetes than women with other blood types. For instance, a study published in the Journal of Diabetes Investigation

indicated that women with blood type AB were more likely than women with blood type O to acquire gestational diabetes. It's crucial to remember that although these studies have discovered links between blood types and diabetes, they do not establish a cause and effect relationship. Both blood type and diabetes risk may be influenced by additional variables. Nevertheless, blood type is only one element that might affect diabetes risk and is not a surefire indicator of who will get the disease.

FIGHTING DIABETES WITH CONVENTIONAL AND BLOOD

Traditional Diabetes Treatment and Blood Sugar Monitoring Techniques

Millions of individuals throughout the world suffer from the chronic disease of diabetes. Diabetes cannot be cured, but it can be effectively treated with a combination of traditional treatments and blood sugar monitoring. We will discuss the many strategies for combating diabetes utilizing these treatments in this article.

Making lifestyle adjustments, taking medication, and forming good habits are the traditional approaches to treating diabetes. Adopting a nutritious diet is one of the most significant lifestyle adjustments that can help control blood sugar levels. This usually entails cutting out on sugary and processed meals while consuming more healthy grains, fruits, vegetables, and lean protein.

Regular exercise is a crucial lifestyle change as well.

Exercise can assist improve insulin sensitivity, lower blood sugar levels, and promote weight loss, all of which can aid with better diabetes management. Furthermore, oral medicines and/or insulin injections may be administered to assist maintain blood sugar levels.

A key component of managing diabetes is blood sugar monitoring in addition to these traditional techniques. Daily monitoring of blood sugar levels can assist persons with diabetes understand how their bodies are responding to various medications and lifestyle modifications. Using this knowledge, dosages of medications or dietary practices can then be changed as necessary.

Blood glucose levels can be checked using a blood glucose meter, continuous glucose monitoring (CGM) systems, or flash glucose monitoring, among other techniques systems. A little drop of blood is used to measure the blood sugar levels with a portable blood glucose meter. On the other hand, CGM devices use a tiny sensor implanted beneath the skin to continually monitor blood sugar levels throughout the day. Rapid glucose monitoring devices take blood sugar readings from the interstitial fluid under the skin using a wearable device.

HOW BEST SUPPLEMENT FOR IMPROVING BLOOD SUGAR

For their potential to lower blood sugar levels in those with diabetes or prediabetes, a number of supplements have been researched. Here are some of the top vitamins and minerals for lowering blood sugar:

1. Alpha-Lipoic Acid (ALA): ALA is an antioxidant that may improve insulin sensitivity and decrease inflammation to lower blood sugar levels. Moreover, it has been demonstrated to lessen diabetic neuropathy symptoms and enhance nerve function.

2. Chromium: is a chemical that aids in the metabolism of glucose. It may increase insulin sensitivity and reduce blood sugar levels in persons with type 2 diabetes, according to studies.

3. Cinnamon: Studies have indicated that cinnamon lowers fasting blood sugar and increases insulin sensitivity. Moreover, it might lower inflammation and raise cholesterol levels.

4. Magnesium: A mineral that aids in the metabolism of glucose. It may increase insulin sensitivity and reduce blood sugar levels in persons with type 2 diabetes, according to studies.

5. Berberine: Research has demonstrated the anti-inflammatory and blood sugar-lowering properties of this plant ingredient.

Moreover, it might increase cholesterol levels and insulin sensitivity.

6 Gymnema Sylvestre: Diabetes has traditionally been treated with the herb gymnema sylvestre. By increasing insulin release and decreasing glucose absorption, it may reduce blood sugar levels.While these supplements could help lower blood sugar levels, it's crucial to remember that they shouldn't be used in place of medical care or a healthy lifestyle. Before taking any new supplements, those who have diabetes or prediabetes also should speak with their doctor.

For their potential to lower blood sugar levels in those with diabetes or prediabetes, a number of supplements have been researched. Here are some of the top vitamins and minerals for lowering blood sugar:

TYPES THERAPIES

There are numerous different therapies that can be used to treat different mental health disorders, and each psychotherapy has its own special methods and strategies. The following are just a few of the most typical therapies:

1. Cognitive behavioral therapy (CBT): CBT is a focused, short-term therapy that assists patients in altering unfavorable beliefs and behaviors. It focuses on how ideas, feelings, and actions are related to one another and how these relationships can be changed to enhance mental health.

2. Psychoanalytic Therapy: Psychoanalytic treatment is a protracted form of therapy that seeks to give patients insight into hidden feelings and thoughts that might be causing their mental health issues. To better understand current behavior, it frequently entails examining past relationships and early experiences.

3. Humanistic therapy: Humanistic therapy places a strong emphasis on self-discovery and self-improvement. It highlights a person's capability for development and self-actualization and promotes accountability and self-awareness.

4. Interpersonal Therapy (IPT): IPT is a brief form of therapy that aims to enhance interpersonal connections. It aids people in recognizing and fixing interpersonal issues that can be a factor in their mental health issues.

5.Dialectical Behavior Therapy (DBT): DBT is a form of therapy that blends mindfulness-based practices, acceptance-based techniques, and cognitive-behavioral procedures. It is frequently used to treat illnesses like borderline personality disorders and others that have trouble controlling their emotions.

6. Psychodynamic Therapy: To assist people in comprehending and altering their behavioral patterns, psychodynamic therapy focuses on the subconscious and prior experiences.

7 Family Therapy: Working alongside family members to solve issues inside the family is a component of the family therapy modality. Families going through difficulties or transitions, including divorce or the addition of a new family member, may find it to be especially useful.

8. Group Therapy: In group therapy, a therapist works with a group of people to address concerns or difficulties that they have in common. It can be especially beneficial for people who gain support and criticism from others.

9. Art Therapy: Art therapy involves the use of art as a vehicle for communication and self-expression. It can be especially beneficial for people who have trouble vocally expressing their emotions.

10. Play Therapy: Treatment approach is the use of play as a tool for self-expression and communication, particularly with young children. It can be especially beneficial for kids who struggle to vocally express themselves.

CHAPTER TWO
DIABETES VERSUS BORDERLINE DIABETES

The ability of the body to control blood sugar levels is a factor in the two distinct illnesses of diabetes and borderline diabetes, commonly referred to as prediabetes.

High blood sugar levels are a defining feature of diabetes, a chronic medical disorder caused by the body's inability to generate or use insulin, a hormone that controls blood sugar. Type 1 diabetes, which results from an autoimmune reaction that kills leptin pancreatic cells, and type 2 diabetes, which is brought on by a mix of genetic and lifestyle factors like weight and inactivity, are the two main kinds of diabetes.

Contrarily, prediabetes is a condition where blood sugar levels are elevated but just not high enough to be classified as diabetes. Prediabetic individuals are more likely to acquire type 2 diabetes in addition to additional health issues like stroke and coronary artery disease.

Despite certain parallels, there are also some significant differences between diabetes and prediabetes. For instance: "Although prediabetes can frequently be reversed with lifestyle modifications such as a greater amount of exercise, weight loss, and healthy eating habits, prediabetes is a chronic illness that requires continuing management.

While prediabetes is frequently diagnosed with a single blood test that examines fasting blood sugar levels or A1C levels, diabetes is typically diagnosed with a blood test that analyzes blood sugar levels over time (a measure of average blood sugar levels over the past 2-3 months).

Individuals with prediabetes may be able to manage their disease by lifestyle modifications alone, whereas persons with diabetes frequently need medication, such as insulin or oral medicines, to control their blood sugar levels.

In order to lower their chance of acquiring type 2 diabetes and other health concerns, people with prediabetes should actively consider their situation and adjust their lifestyle. Blood sugar levels and any associated health issues should be closely managed by diabetics in collaboration with their healthcare providers.

Diabetes Types 1 vs. Diabetes Types 2?

Type 1 and type 2 diabetes both affect how the body handles blood sugar, but they are chronic illnesses with different underlying causes and call for different treatment modalities. The following are some significant parallels and variances between type 1 and type 2 diabetes:

Similarities:

Both types of diabetes are characterized by issues with insulin, a hormone that controls the body's blood sugar levels.

In both types of diabetes, high blood sugar levels can result in long-term problems include kidney damage, nerve damage, and cardiovascular disease.

Both types of diabetics may have symptoms like excessive thirst, frequent urination, and exhaustion.

Differences: Type 1 diabetes is an autoimmune condition in which the body attacks and kills the cells that produce insulin in the pancreas, leaving the body deficient in insulin. Contrarily, type 2 diabetes is a metabolic condition in which the body stops producing enough insulin or grows resistant to its effects.

While type 2 diabetes is commonly discovered in adulthood and is frequently linked to obesity and a sedentary lifestyle, type 1 diabetes is normally discovered in childhood or adolescent.

Insulin therapy is used to treat type 1 diabetes, although type 2 diabetes can frequently be controlled with dietary and activity changes as well as drugs that improve the body's ability to utilise insulin.

While ketoacidosis, a potentially fatal illness brought on by an accumulation of ketones in the blood, is uncommon in type 2 diabetes, it is more common in people with type 1 diabetes.

Type 1 diabetes cannot be avoided, however good lifestyle choices can frequently delay or prevent type 2 diabetes.

While there are some obvious differences between type 1 and type 2 diabetes, it's crucial to keep in mind that there can also be some overlap and variance within each kind. It's crucial to get medical attention if you have concerns about your blood sugar levels or diabetes risk factors because both types of diabetes can have major health repercussions if left untreated.

CHAPTER THREE
CAUSES OF DIABETES

High blood sugar levels are a defining feature of diabetes, a chronic metabolic illness caused by the body's inability to make or utilize insulin. Diabetes has a number of root causes, including:

1.Genetics: The likelihood of acquiring diabetes is increased by a family history of the disease.

2. Lifestyle factors: Type 2 diabetes can develop as a result of poor diet, insufficient exercise, and also being overweight or obese.

3. Insulin resistance: When the body's cells lose their receptivity to insulin, it is more

challenging for glucose to get to the cells and be utilised as fuel.

4. Autoimmune factors: Type 1 diabetes results in a lack of insulin production because the immune system targets and kills the pancreatic cells that produce insulin.

5. Pancreatic disease or damage: In some circumstances, pancreatic disease or damage can prevent the pancreas from producing insulin, which can result in the onset of diabetes.

6. Medications: Certain drugs, like corticosteroids and antipsychotics, can make you more likely to get diabetes.

7. Gestational diabetes: Some pregnant women experience this condition, which often goes away after delivery. Yet, women

who have gestational diabetes are more likely to eventually develop type 2 diabetes. Overall, there are many different factors that contribute to the development of diabetes, making the disease's causes complicated and multiple.

WHAT TO EAT AND WHEN TO EAT IT TO AVOID DIABETES

Diabetes is a chronic condition that interferes with the body's ability to process blood sugar (glucose). A healthy diet and way of life can help manage blood sugar levels and lower the chance of getting diabetes, even though no one food or diet can completely prevent or cure diabetes.

These are some sophisticated suggestions on eating to prevent diabetes:

1. Put an emphasis on whole, nutrient-dense foods: Go for foods high in fiber and nutrients, such as fruits, vegetables, whole grains, legumes, and lean proteins. These foods contain important vitamins and minerals while also assisting in blood sugar regulation.

2. Steer clear of highly processed foods. Highly processed foods frequently contain added sugars, refined carbs, and unhealthy fats that can increase insulin resistance and the risk of developing diabetes. Restrict or stay away from things like packaged snacks, sugary beverages, and fast food.

3. Go for healthy fats: Healthy fats, such those in nuts, seeds, avocados, and fatty fish,

can enhance insulin sensitivity and lessen inflammation. Fats are calorie-dense, therefore it's still necessary to eat them in moderation.

4. Be mindful of portion sizes: Eating too much can result in weight gain, which is a significant risk factor for diabetes. Reduce the size of your plates and eat mindfully to help manage portion proportions

5. Drink in moderation: Alcohol intake can result in elevated blood sugar levels and raise the risk of getting diabetes. If you decide to consume alcohol, do it moderately and with meals.

6. Speak with a trained dietitian: If you are at risk for developing diabetes or have a family history of the disease, speaking with a registered dietitian can help you design a

specific nutrition plan to control your blood sugar levels and lower your risk.

ADVANCED TOPIC ON EATING TIMES TO REDUCE RISK OF DIABETES

Diabetes is a chronic illness that interferes with the body's ability to process glucose, a form of sugar. The body converts carbs to glucose after a meal, which is subsequently used as fuel.

This process is compromised in diabetics, either as a result of insufficient insulin production by the body or insulin resistance in the body's cells. As a result, blood glucose levels rise, which can cause a number of health issues.

The timing of your meals may have an impact on your risk of diabetes, according to some data. In example, having a heavy meal in the evening, especially one that is high in carbohydrates, may raise your chance of developing diabetes, according to study. This is due to the fact that eating a substantial meal late at night can result in higher blood sugar levels since your body is less able to digest the glucose.

On the other hand, there's some evidence to support the idea that having a heavier meal earlier in the day and a lighter supper in the evening may assist to lower your risk of acquiring diabetes. This is due to the fact that eating earlier in the day gives your body more time to absorb the glucose and can lower your risk of experiencing blood sugar spikes.Although the timing of your meals may affect your likelihood of getting diabetes, there are a number of other factors to take into account as well, including your general diet, exercise routine, and genetics. It's constantly a good idea to discuss your diabetes risk with your healthcare practitioner, who can work with you to create a specialized plan for doing so.

CHAPTER FOUR

DANGER THAT LURK BEYOND CALORIES AND CARBS BEYOND CALORIES AND CARBS

While calories and carbs are crucial components in determining how to maintain a balanced diet, there are additional hazards that exist. Here are a few illustrations:

1. Nutritional deficits can result from focusing just on calorie and carb intake and overlooking other vital nutrients like

vitamins, minerals, and fiber that our bodies require. This may result in nutrient shortages, which may result in a variety of medical issues.

2. Food additives: A lot of processed foods contain ingredients like preservatives, colors, and flavorings that could be bad for our health. Several of these additives have been connected to allergies, cancer, and other health problems.

3. Foodborne illnesses: Eating food that has been tainted or incorrectly stored can result in food poisoning, which can be extremely sickening or even fatal. In order to reduce the chance of contracting a foodborne illness, it is crucial to use proper food preparation and handling methods.

4. Environmental poisons: Certain meals may include chemicals, heavy metals, or other environmental toxins that can build up in our bodies over time and harm our health.

5. Emotional eating: Using food as a coping mechanism for stress, worry, or other emotional problems can result in unhealthful eating patterns and weight gain. Finding healthy ways to cope with stress and emotions is crucial, as is addressing the underlying causes of emotional eating.

It's crucial to remember that eating a balanced diet entails more than just keeping track of your calories and carbs. For optimum health and wellbeing, a balanced diet consisting of a variety of nutrient-dense foods is necessary, as are healthy lifestyle practices including frequent exercise and stress reduction.

A SIMPLE WAY TO STOP EATING

For the purpose of reaching and maintaining a healthy weight, appetite control is crucial. Nonetheless, many people find it difficult to control their appetite. It's crucial to keep in mind that cutting back on food doesn't mean you have to go without or deny yourself of necessary nutrients. In this project, we'll talk about some quick and simple techniques for controlling your hunger without making you feel famished or deprived

1. Drink Plenty of Water: Water consumption is a simple and efficient strategy to reduce appetite. We frequently

eat too much because we misinterpret our appetite for being hungry. You can consume less calories by drinking water before meals to make you feel satisfied. Try to consume 8 to 10 glasses of water daily.

2. Consume high-fiber foods: Fiber-rich foods can keep you feeling fuller for longer. Foods high in fiber and low in calories, such as fruits, vegetables, whole grains, and legumes, are the best options for persons trying to curb their hunger.Moreover, fiber slows down digestion, which helps control blood sugar levels and keeps you fuller for longer.

3. Consume Enough Protein: Protein is a food that requires more time to digest, making it a good choice for keeping you feeling fuller for longer. Eat foods high in

protein, such as eggs, lean meat, chicken, fish, beans, and legumes, as part of your diet. You may lessen cravings, curb your appetite, and lose weight by eating these items.

4. Engage in Mindful Eating: Mindful eating is the practice of being mindful of your food and eating patterns. It makes you more conscious of your eating habits, ideas, and emotions, which might aid in appetite management. Eat slowly, chew your meal completely, and steer clear of distractions while you're eating, such as the TV or your phone.

5.Get Enough Sleep: Sleep deprivation can interfere with the hormones that control your appetite and satiety, making it harder to limit your food consumption. To control these hormones and lessen hunger sensations, attempt to get a minimum of 7-8 hours of rest each night. Establishing a regular sleep schedule, abstaining from caffeine and gadgets before bed, and creating a peaceful sleeping environment are all examples of good sleep hygiene practices.

6.Stay away from processed foods: These meals tend to be high in calories, sugar, and harmful fats, which might cause you to feel hungry even after you've eaten enough calories. Steer clear of processed foods, such as sodas with added sugar, chips, and fast food.Choose whole foods instead, such as fresh produce, lean meats, and whole grains.

7.Staying active can help you control your appetite and lessen cravings. Your body releases endorphins during exercise, which can help lower stress and maintain mood. You can use these advantages to manage your calorie intake and choose healthier foods

CHAPTER FIVE

SYMPTOM OF DIABETES

Millions of individuals worldwide suffer with diabetes, a long-term metabolic condition. Due to the body's inability to make enough insulin or utilise it effectively, it is characterized by high blood sugar levels. Diabetes can cause severe health issues, such as heart disease, nerve damage, renal disease, and blindness. For an early diagnosis and treatment of diabetes, it is essential to recognize the symptoms. The signs of diabetes will be thoroughly covered in this project effort.

Other people may not experience any symptoms at all, and the signs and symptoms of diabetes might differ from person to person. The most typical signs of diabetes, however, include:

1. Frequent urination: Diabetics may have frequent urine needs, especially at night. This is due to the body's attempt to remove extra sugar from the blood by urinating.

2. Increased thirst: Those with diabetes may experience increased thirst due to frequent urination, which can cause dehydration.

3. Hunger pangs: Those with diabetes may experience increased hunger, even after eating, as a result of the body's inability to utilise glucose properly.

4. Fatigue: Those with diabetes who have high blood sugar levels may experience fatigue and lethargy.

5. Distorted vision: Diabetes can alter the eye's lens, which can impair eyesight.

6.Slow wound healing: The body's capacity to heal wounds and injuries might be hampered by high blood sugar levels.

7.Numbness and tingling in the hands and feet: Diabetes can harm the nerves in the hands and feet, causing numbness and tingling feelings.

8.Weight loss: When the body breaks down fat and muscle tissue for energy, people with type 1 diabetes may have unexplained weight loss.

9. Dry skin and mouth: Dehydration brought on by diabetes might result in dry skin and mouth.

It is significant to remember that diabetes symptoms can appear gradually and may be confused with those of other diseases. If you have any of the aforementioned symptoms, it is imperative to see a doctor, especially if you have a family history of diabetes or other risk factors like obesity or a sedentary lifestyle.

DIABETES COMPLICATION

Introduction: Millions of individuals throughout the world suffer from the chronic disease of diabetes. It is brought on by the body's inability to make or utilise insulin, a hormone that controls blood sugar levels. Over time, having elevated levels of sugar in your blood can result in a variety of health issues, some of which can be fatal. The most prevalent diabetes complications, their signs and symptoms, and therapies will all be covered in this project.

1. Cardiovascular Disease: The major cause of death for diabetics is cardiovascular disease. Blood arteries can get damaged by high blood sugar levels, which also raises the risk of heart attack and stroke. Chest pain, shortness of breath, and numbness or weakness in the arms or legs are all signs of cardiovascular disease. In addition to lifestyle modifications including diet and exercise, treatment options may include

medications to decrease blood pressure and cholesterol levels.

2. Neuropathy: Diabetics may experience neuropathy, a form of nerve damage. The feet and legs are the areas it most frequently affects, and symptoms including tingling, numbness, and burning pain are prevalent. Neuropathy occasionally also affects the hands and arms. In addition to lifestyle modifications like giving up smoking and managing blood sugar levels, treatment options may also include medication to treat pain and enhance nerve function.

3. Retinopathy: Diabetics who suffer from retinopathy experience eye problems. High blood sugar levels harm the blood vessels in the retina, the area of the eye that is important for vision, causing it to happen.

Blurred vision,floaters and trouble seeing in dim lighting. Medication to control the levels of sugar in the blood and laser treatment to stop future retinal damage are possible forms of treatment.

4. Nephropathy: Diabetics may experience nephropathy, a form of kidney injury. It happens when elevated levels of glucose in the blood harm the veins and arteries in the kidneys, resulting in either poor or complete renal failure. Swelling of something like the hands, feet, or face, as well as extreme urination and frequent urination, are possible symptoms. In addition to lifestyle modifications like cutting back on salt intake and stopping smoking, treatment options may include medications to control your blood pressure and sugar levels.

PREVENTION AND TREATING DIABETES

Millions of individuals around the world suffer from the chronic medical illness known as diabetes. It is characterized by high blood sugar levels as a result of the body's inability to make or use insulin, a hormone that controls blood sugar levels, appropriately. Serious health issues like heart disease, renal failure, and blindness can develop as a result of diabetes. But diabetes is preventable, and the earlier it is identified, the simpler it is to control.

This research will cover a variety of diabetes prevention strategies, such as dietary changes, lifestyle adjustments, and routine physical examinations. We'll also look at the impact that education and awareness have in managing and preventing diabetes.

changes to one's way of life

Making lifestyle changes is one of the most effective methods to prevent diabetes. Increasing physical exercise, maintaining a healthy weight, and abstaining from tobacco use are all part of this. Regular exercise can help manage blood sugar levels and increase insulin sensitivity. A minimum of 150 minutes of moderate-intensity aerobic activity each week, distributed over at least three days, is advised by the American Diabetes Association. Moreover, muscle mass can be increased through resistance exercise, which enhances insulin sensitivity. Keeping a healthy weight is essential for avoiding diabetes. Obesity or being overweight can enhance the risk of acquiring diabetes by 80%. A good diet and consistent exercise can assist people in achieving and maintaining a healthy weight.

The Mediterranean diet and the Dietary Approaches to Stop Hypertension (DASH) are two examples of healthy eating regimens that have been demonstrated to lower the risk of diabetes.

Another significant risk factor for diabetes is tobacco usage. Smoking makes people more insulin resistant, which can lead to type 2 diabetes. Giving up smoking can help lower your risk of getting diabetes and enhance your general health.

Nutritional alterations: In addition to lifestyle adjustments, dietary improvements can aid in the prevention of diabetes. Lean proteins, healthy fats, and a variety of fruits, vegetables, whole grains should all be present in a nutritious diet. Limit your intake of foods that are heavy in sugar, saturated and trans fats, and processed carbs. A measure of how quickly a diet elevates blood sugar levels is called the glycemic index (GI). White bread and sweetened beverages are examples of foods with a high GI that can elevate blood sugar levels and increase the risk of developing diabetes. Low GI foods, such whole grains and legumes, can help control blood sugar levels and lower the risk of developing diabetes.

regular medical examinations

The prevention and control of diabetes depend heavily on routine medical examinations. Those who are at a high risk of acquiring diabetes, such as those who are obese, have a family history of the disease, or have a sedentary lifestyle, should undergo routine diabetes screenings.A measure of how quickly a diet elevates blood sugar levels is called the glycemic index (GI). White bread and sweetened beverages are examples of foods with a high GI that can elevate blood sugar levels and increase the risk of developing diabetes. Low GI foods, such whole grains and legumes, can help control blood sugar levels and lower the risk of developing diabetes.

REGULAR MEDICAL EXAMINATIONS

The prevention and control of diabetes depend heavily on routine medical examinations. Those who are at a high risk of acquiring diabetes, such as those who are obese, have a family history of the disease, or have a sedentary lifestyle, should undergo routine diabetes screenings.

TREATMENT OF DIABETES

Lifestyle Modifications: Changing one's way of life is the first procedure for managing diabetes. This entails altering your eating habits and upping your physical activity. A nutritious diet low in sugar, salt, and saturated fat can aid with blood sugar regulation. Regular exercise is essential for regulating blood sugar levels and preserving a healthy weight. Exercise also increases glycemic control, which can improve how well the body uses insulin.

Prescription drugs can be used if lifestyle modifications alone are insufficient to regulate blood sugar levels. To treat diabetes, a variety of drugs are available. They consist of:

1. Metformin: The first drug typically administered for type 2 diabetes is metformin. It functions by reducing the liver's output of glucose and raising the body's sensitivity to insulin.

2. Sulfonylureas: A class of drugs known as sulfonylureas encourages the pancreas to produce more insulin.

3. DPP-4 inhibitors: DPP-4 inhibitors act by boosting pancreatic production of insulin while reducing hepatic production of glucose.

4. GLP-1 receptor agonists: GLP-1 receptor agonists function by boosting the synthesis of insulin and reducing the amount of glucose the liver produces. Also, they aid in slowing down food digestion, which can aid with blood sugar regulation.

5. SGLT2 inhibitors: SGLT2 inhibitors reduce blood sugar levels by preventing the kidneys from reabsorbing glucose.

6. Insulin Therapy: Insulin therapy may be administered if medication is insufficient to regulate blood sugar levels. The pancreas produces the hormone insulin, which aids in controlling blood sugar levels. To assist control blood sugar levels, insulin is injected into the body as part of insulin therapy. In addition to rapid-acting insulin, there are also short-acting, intermediate-acting, and long-acting insulins. Depending on the person's requirements and the extent of their diabetes, the type of insulin given will vary.

Surgery: Surgery for the management of diabetes may be advised in specific circumstances. Typically, those with type 2 diabetes and significant obesity who have failed to regulate their blood glucose levels through previous treatments should only consider this. For the treatment of diabetes, bypass surgery for the stomach and head of the pancreas diversion surgery are the two main surgical procedures. Reduced stomach size and/or bypassing of a portion of the small intestine as a result of these operations can help control blood sugar levels.

CONCLUSION

Millions of individuals throughout the world suffer from the chronic disease of diabetes. It is a disorder that requires continual management, such as dietary adjustments and drug administration. Many problems, such as cardiovascular disease, kidney failure, nerve damage, and blindness, can be brought on by diabetes. However, many of these consequences can be avoided or postponed with careful management and blood sugar level control.A comprehensive strategy that incorporates frequent blood sugar testing, a nutritious diet, regular exercise, and medication management is the key to treating diabetes. Metformin, sulfonylureas, DPP-4 inhibitors, GLP-1 receptor agonists, SGLT2 inhibitors, and insulin therapy are a few of the drug kinds that are used to treat diabetes. The ideal pharmaceutical regimen for your particular needs should be decided in close consultation with your healthcare professional.

Moreover, diabetes education and awareness are essential for managing and preventing the disease.Individuals with diabetes should be informed about their illness, comprehend the need of adopting healthy lifestyle habits and managing their medications, and seek assistance when necessary. To help their loved ones manage the disease, family members and carers should also receive diabetes education.

In conclusion, diabetes must be continuously managed and cared for as a significant health disease. Individuals who have diabetes can live healthy, productive lives with adequate care. It is crucial to adopt a thorough strategy that incorporates pharmaceutical treatment, healthy lifestyle choices, and informational and awareness campaigns regarding the condition. We may treat and prevent the negative effects of diabetes by cooperating.

9 798391 534068